DON'T **DIVORCE** YET

A Practical Guide To Save Your Marriage And Rebuild Relationship With Love, Peace, Understanding, Values And Trust

Beverly Conner

Copyright © [2024] [Beverly Conner]

All Rights Reserved

CONTENTS

Introduction

Marriage could be a rough ride or an easy one. At the beginning, everything feels effortless. There's laughter, passion, and a deep sense of connection. But as time passes, life gets in the way—stress, misunderstandings, and unmet expectations pile up. Suddenly, the person you once couldn't imagine living without now feels like a stranger.

For many couples, this moment of disconnection leads to an unbearable question: Is it time to walk away? Divorce starts to feel like the only way to escape the pain. After all, how do you rebuild trust after so many arguments? How do you reignite love when the fire feels long extinguished?

But before you give up, ask yourself this: What if there's still hope?

This book isn't about dismissing the challenges in your relationship. It's not about pretending the pain doesn't exist or forcing you to stay in a situation where you're miserable. Instead, it offers you a chance—a structured, heartfelt 30-day journey to rediscover what brought you together in the first place and rebuild the bond that feels so broken now.

No one enters a marriage expecting it to fail. You promised to love, honor, and cherish each other, and you meant it. But over time, cracks began to form. Maybe it was the little things at first—a sarcastic comment, a missed anniversary or even lack of understanding. Over time, those little cracks became deeper, forming walls that now feel impossible to tear down.

Perhaps your communication broke down. Maybe trust was shattered. Maybe someone cheated Or maybe the pressures of daily life (work, kids, finances) pushed you further apart. Whatever the cause, the pain is real. And yet, love isn't something that just disappears. It's still there, buried under the hurt, waiting for a chance to resurface.

This book isn't a quick fix or a miracle cure. It's a step-by-step guide to help you rebuild your marriage, one day at a time. Over the next 30 days, you'll focus on simple, meaningful actions that can bring healing, trust, and intimacy back into your relationship.

These aren't grand, expensive gestures. They're small, deliberate acts of love: planning a surprise date night, cooking a favorite meal, writing a heartfelt note, or simply listening without interrupting. Each day, you'll be encouraged to set aside your pride and pain and choose love even when it feels impossible.

You might be thinking, Why should I be the one to make all the effort? That's a fair question, especially if your partner has hurt you deeply. But love has a way of transforming things. When you lead with kindness and vulnerability, you create an environment where healing can take place. It's not about doing everything perfectly;

it's about showing up with an open heart and a willingness to try.

Over the years, I've seen marriages that seemed beyond saving find their way back to love. I've seen couples who were barely speaking start to laugh together again. I've seen relationships where trust was shattered and rebuilt stronger than ever.

There's one story that stands out for me– a couple who had already started drafting their divorce papers. They couldn't have a conversation without it turning into a fight. They were convinced they were better off apart. Out of desperation, they decided to give a 30-day challenge like this one a try.

The first few days were awkward. They didn't trust each other's intentions, and the resentment ran deep. But they kept at it. Slowly, the walls between them began to crumble. By the end of the challenge, they weren't just tolerating each other; they were holding hands, planning their future, and rediscovering the love they thought was gone.

Their story isn't unique. Countless couples have found that, with effort and commitment, it's possible to rekindle the love that brought them together.

As you go through this book, you'll be guided through thirty days of intentional love. Each day focuses on a simple but powerful act of kindness, connection, or vulnerability. Some days will be easier than others, and there will be times when you feel like giving up. That's normal.

This journey is more than saving your marriage—it's about rediscovering the best parts of yourself and your relationship. You'll learn how to communicate, forgive, and show love in ways that create lasting change.

Even if your partner doesn't seem approachable when you start, your efforts can set the stage for transformation. Love has a ripple effect, and sometimes all it takes is one person to lead the way.

Divorce might seem like the easiest option right now. It promises relief from the pain and conflict. But before you take that step, consider this: the love you once shared is still worth fighting for. Your marriage doesn't have to end in heartbreak. It can become a story of resilience, forgiveness, and renewed connection.

These next thirty days could change everything. They could help you tear down the walls that have kept you apart and build something stronger in their place. All it takes is a willingness to try, one day at a time.

Your marriage isn't over. Not yet. And if you're willing to take this journey, you might just find that the best is yet to come.

PART ONE: Small Gestures, Big impacts.

DAY 1

A Heartfelt Message

This is the beginning of your journey to rebuild what feels broken, to rediscover the connection you once cherished with your spouse. It may feel overwhelming to take the first step, especially if you're carrying pain, resentment, or exhaustion. But love begins with a single act, and today's challenge is simple yet profoundly powerful: write a heartfelt message to your spouse and leave it on the dinner table or bed.

You may hesitate at the thought of this. Perhaps you're thinking, Why should I make the first move? They've hurt me too. Or maybe you feel unsure about what to say, worried that your words will fall on deaf ears. But this is not about expecting anything in return. It's about choosing to lead with love, even when it feels hard.

Think back to the moments that made you fall in love. What was it about your spouse that made your heart race? Was it their kindness, their sense of humor, or the way they made you feel safe? Those qualities are still there, even if they've been overshadowed by time and challenges.

Take a quiet moment today. Find a pen and paper, and let your heart guide your words. This isn't about writing a perfect letter; it's about writing an honest one. Start with something simple. Express gratitude for something they've done recently, even if it's small. Remind them of a happy memory you shared. Let them know you still see them, even through the hurt.

For example, you might write:

"I know things have been difficult between us lately, and there's so much I wish I could change. But I want you to know that I still care deeply for you. I remember the way we used to talk for hours, dreaming about the future. Those memories remind me of how much we've shared and how much I value you. Thank you for all that you do for our family, even when it feels unnoticed. I'm committed to working through this with you, one step at a time."

It doesn't have to be long or poetic; it just needs to come from your heart. Once you've written your message, place it somewhere they'll find it, in a place that feels intimate and thoughtful. The dinner table, where you've shared countless meals. The bed, where you've shared your most vulnerable moments.

This small act may feel insignificant, but its impact can be profound. Your words have the power to soften their heart, to remind them that love still lingers between you. They may not respond right away, and that's okay. This is the beginning of something bigger, it's a journey of rebuilding, one loving act at a time.

Take a deep breath, write your message, and trust the process. Today, you are choosing love over pride, hope over despair. And that choice is the first step toward healing.

DAY 2

The Words That Leave Scars

Words are powerful. They can build bridges or burn them to the ground. In marriage, they hold the potential to nurture love or cause wounds that may never fully heal. Today's focus is on protecting your relationship by being mindful of what you say. We'll explore ten phrases that should never be spoken to your spouse, no matter how frustrated or hurt you feel. These words don't just express temporary emotions; they cut deep and often leave scars that linger long after the moment has passed.

When you're angry, words can fly out before you've had the chance to think. But those words, once spoken, can't be taken back. They hang in the air, seeping into your spouse's heart, carrying weight you might not have intended. Even when arguments fade, hurtful words have a way of staying alive, playing over and over in the mind of the person who heard them.

Here are ten things you should never say to your spouse and why they can be so damaging:

I regret being with you; *This phrase strikes at the very core of your relationship. It invalidates all the love, memories, and effort you've shared. It makes your spouse feel like they were a mistake, a decision you wish you could undo. Words like this destroy trust and create a sense of worthlessness.*

You're not like my ex; *Comparing your spouse to someone from your past is like telling them they don't measure up. It plants seeds of insecurity and resentment. Your spouse should never feel like they are competing with a ghost from your past.*

You always ruin everything; *This sentence is a dagger. It exaggerates faults and disregards the good things your spouse* *does. It paints them as perpetually flawed, leaving no room for understanding or forgiveness.*

You're overreacting; *Dismissing your spouse's feelings as exaggerated or invalid is a surefire way to make them feel unheard and unimportant. Everyone's emotions are valid, even if you don't fully understand them.*

I wish I never married you; *This statement cuts deeper than most. It erases the foundation of your relationship and makes your spouse feel disposable. Even said in anger, it leaves wounds that take years to heal if they ever do.*

You're just like your mother/father; *This is often said with a negative connotation, turning a loved one's family traits into a weapon. It's a deeply personal attack, implying that they've inherited flaws they can't escape.*

You'll never change; *This phrase shuts the door to growth and improvement. It tells your spouse that no matter how hard they try, they'll never be good enough in your eyes.*

I don't care anymore: *Indifference is often more painful than anger. This phrase signals the withdrawal of love, making your spouse feel abandoned and unloved.*

You're not good at anything*: Criticizing someone's abilities or worth can crush their spirit. It's not just about the specific insult but the message that they have no value in your eyes.*

You'll never make me happy*: Happiness in marriage is a shared responsibility, not a one-person job. This statement unfairly places the blame on your spouse, making them feel like they're failing in the relationship.*

Words have the power to shape how we see ourselves and our relationships. In marriage, hurtful words don't just wound in the moment; they leave behind scars that alter the way your spouse feels about you and themselves. These scars can fester into insecurity, resentment, and a loss of trust.

When you speak carelessly, it tells your spouse that their feelings don't matter. It creates an emotional distance that grows with every hurtful word. Over time, this distance becomes harder to bridge, and the relationship suffers. Think about it: when was the last time your spouse said something that hurt you? Can you still hear those words in your mind? That's the power of language. And while hurtful words can break a bond, kind words can rebuild it.

Today's challenge is not just about avoiding hurtful words but about replacing them with healing ones. When you feel anger bubbling up, pause. Take a deep breath. Instead of reacting with words that tear down, choose words that build up. For example, instead of saying, "You always ruin everything," you could say, "I'm feeling frustrated right now, but I want us to work through this together."

Every word you speak has the potential to either damage or strengthen your marriage. Choose to speak life into your relationship. Be the partner who uplifts, reassures, and nurtures love with your words.

Remember that your voice carries immense power in your spouse's life. Use it wisely, and let it be a tool for healing and connection.

DAY 3

Letting go of anger and resentment

Today, I want to ask you for something that might feel incredibly difficult: to commit to a fresh start with an open mind. This is not about pretending the past didn't happen or erasing the pain you've endured. It's about choosing to let go of the grip the past has on your heart so that you can create a new future for your marriage.

Holding onto anger and resentment may feel justified. After all, the hurt you've experienced is real. But as long as you hold onto the pain, it will continue to shape your thoughts, your words, and your actions. It will become the lens through which you see your partner. That lens, clouded by past mistakes, will make it nearly impossible to see the possibility of something better.

Letting go isn't easy. There will be moments when memories of arguments, broken promises, or disappointments resurface. You might feel anger bubbling up, questioning why you should even bother trying. But in those moments, remind yourself that holding onto pain is not the same as protecting yourself. It's only weighing you down.

Think about when your marriage began to feel different. When did things start to shift? Was it a specific argument, a pattern of neglect, or something unspoken that grew over time? Reflect on these moments—not to assign blame, but to better understand the cracks that formed in your relationship. Awareness is the first step to healing.

Maybe it was small things at first. A harsh word is spoken in frustration. A busy schedule that left little time for connection. The excitement of early love gave way to the exhaustion of daily life, and without realizing it, you both began to drift apart. Recognizing these moments isn't about dwelling on them; it's about learning from them. What went unsaid? What actions hurt without words?

And most importantly, what could be done differently now?

Committing to a fresh start means deciding to see your partner as they are today, not as they were in the moments that hurt you. It means choosing forgiveness, even if it feels undeserved, not because they've earned it, but because you deserve the freedom it brings.

Forgiveness doesn't excuse the hurt, nor does it mean you won't feel the sting of past wounds. But forgiveness is a gift you give yourself—a way of saying, I won't let this pain control my heart any longer. When you let go of the past, you make space for love, understanding, and the possibility of something better.

Today, take a moment to reflect on what a fresh start could look like. What would it mean to approach your partner with an open mind, free from the weight of past mistakes? This doesn't mean ignoring problems; it means addressing them with hope rather than resentment.

You can't change what's been done, but you can choose how to move forward. And today, with courage and an open heart, you're taking the first step.

DAY 4

A Meal Made with Love

Love is simple, yet deeply meaningful: prepare your spouse's favorite meal and set the table for them. This is more than just cooking; it's an expression of care, a quiet way of saying, I see you, and I still cherish you.

Food has a unique power to connect us. Think about the memories you've created around meals—the laughter shared over dinner, the quiet comfort of breakfast together, the joy of discovering each other's favorite dishes. Preparing a meal for someone isn't just about nourishment; it's about love, effort, and thoughtfulness.

When you take the time to prepare your spouse's favorite dish, you're sending them a message: I remember you. I know what you love. I care enough to make something special for you. Even if the relationship feels strained right now, this act can begin to soften the edges.

Set the table with intention. Don't just toss plates and utensils down—make it inviting. Light a candle, use the good dishes, or add a small touch like a folded napkin. These small details show effort, and effort is love made visible.

It's natural to hope your spouse will notice and appreciate this gesture. Maybe they'll smile, thank you, and enjoy every bite. But what if they don't? What if they barely acknowledge it, or worse, seem indifferent? It's important to prepare your heart for this possibility.

This act of love is not about their reaction but your intention. Love, at its purest, is given freely, without expectation. If your spouse doesn't respond the way you hoped, don't let it discourage you. Take a deep breath, relax, and remind yourself that this is just one step in a larger journey. Healing and rebuilding take time, and every small act adds up, even if it's not immediately visible.

If your spouse asks why you're doing this, respond gently and warmly. You might say, "I remembered you love this dish," or "It's been a long time since we had this together." These responses are simple and kind, leaving room for connection without pressure.

Acts of love like this can rekindle memories of better times. Even if your spouse doesn't openly express it, the effort you've put in will leave an impression. It shows them that, despite everything, you're willing to try—that the bond you share still matters to you.

While you serve the meal, take a moment to appreciate the significance of what you're doing. You're creating space for connection, warmth, and maybe even the first spark of renewed intimacy. Whether they say it or not, your love will be felt.Remember, this is not about perfection. It's about showing up with a willing heart. One meal may not heal everything, but it's a start. And every start is a step closer to the love you're working to rebuild.

DAY 5

The Magic of Little actions

You will focus on the power of small, thoughtful actions that can breathe life back into your relationship. Love isn't always about grand declarations or sweeping gestures; sometimes, it's found in the quiet moments that show, I care about you. You matter to me.

Start the day by planting a soft kiss on your spouse's forehead or cheek as they wake up. This simple act can communicate tenderness without words. It's a gesture that says, I see you, and I want to start the day with love. If they're surprised or even caught off guard, that's okay. You're breaking through the usual routines, and sometimes love feels unexpected.

After that, do something thoughtful. Maybe it's making them coffee or preparing breakfast. It doesn't have to be elaborate; the effort itself speaks volumes. A cup of coffee prepared just the way they like it can be a small yet meaningful way to show you're thinking of them.

As the day unfolds, look for an opportunity to surprise them with a little gift. It could be something as simple as their favorite ice cream, a bouquet, or a bottle of wine. If you know there's something they enjoy—a snack, a book, or even a small trinket, get it for them. These gestures may seem small, but they have the power to touch the heart.

If your spouse asks why you're doing this, smile warmly. Give them a peck on the cheek and say, "Because I love you." Let those words linger, simple yet profound. You don't need a grand explanation; love, after all, is reason enough.

But what if they don't respond the way you hope? What if they seem indifferent, dismissive, or even reject the gift? This can be disheartening, but I want you to remember that this journey is not about instant results. It's about planting seeds. Love is a process, not a transaction. Your efforts may not bear fruit immediately, but they are building something over time.

When you show consistent care, even in the face of rejection, you're creating a space for healing. You're gently and patiently reminding your partner that love still exists between you. Every small gesture is a brick in the foundation you're rebuilding.

The magic of little gestures lies in their ability to pierce through walls that have built up over time. They remind your partner of the kindness, thoughtfulness, and care that may have been overshadowed by the struggles of daily life. These actions say, without words, I'm here. I haven't given up on us.

PART TWO: Rekindling Romance

DAY 6

The Date Night

Tonight is about creating a moment of connection, a chance to step away from the daily grind and the tension that may have crept into your relationship. A quiet, thoughtful evening can do wonders to reset the tone between you and your partner. This is the perfect opportunity to plan a cosy date night at home—a simple yet powerful gesture that can rekindle the warmth you once shared.

Start by choosing something you both used to enjoy together: a favorite movie, a beloved TV series, a fun board game, or even a playlist of songs that bring back memories. If you're unsure, pick something your partner loves, even if it's not your personal favorite. The goal is to create a space where they feel seen, valued, and appreciated.

Call your partner gently. Use a soft, inviting tone to draw them in. You could say, "It's been so long since we had a movie night at home," or "I've set something up in the living room—I think you'll enjoy it." These words carry no pressure, just an open invitation to share a moment.
If they respond positively and join you, that's wonderful. Sit together, enjoy the popcorn, and let the shared experience work it's quiet magic. But if they seem reluctant, dismissive, or uninterested, don't let it discourage you. It's easy to feel hurt in such moments but remember that this journey is about consistency and patience.

Go ahead with your plan. Watch the movie, play the game, or enjoy the show on your own. Prepare the popcorn, dim the lights, and make it an enjoyable experience for yourself. Your partner may remain distant for now, but the effort you've put in won't go unnoticed.

Sometimes, curiosity works in your favor. As they hear the laughter from the TV or catch a glimpse of you relaxing and enjoying yourself, they might start to wonder. Why are they doing this? Why are they trying, even after everything? This quiet pondering can spark something deep within—a reflection on their own choices and habits, and perhaps a shift in how they see your efforts.

Love isn't about forcing someone to respond the way you want. It's about showing up, being present, and offering kindness even when it feels unreciprocated. Tonight's date night is an investment in the bond you're rebuilding. Whether they join you or not, you're planting seeds of care and consistency.

Keep your heart open and your expectations light. Trust that small gestures like this, repeated over time, can create ripples of change. Even if tonight doesn't unfold as you hoped, you've taken another step toward reconciling love. Sometimes, the effort alone is enough to spark a change, and one day, they might look back and remember this quiet, thoughtful evening as a moment when love was reignit

DAY 7

A Gentle Reminder Of Love

Small but meaningful act that has the power to reach deep into your partner's heart. a love note. Find a quiet moment and write a simple, heartfelt message. It doesn't need to be long or overly poetic; sincerity is what matters most. Write something like, "I thought of you today and wanted to remind you how much you mean to me," or "You're always in my heart, and I'm so grateful for you." Tuck this note into their bag, lunch box, or somewhere they'll find it unexpectedly during the day.

As they go about their day, this little surprise will remind them that love still exists between you, even in the smallest gestures. It might catch them off guard, or it might bring a smile to their face when they least expect it. Either way, it's a quiet way of saying, I care for you, even now.

Later in the day, reach out with a call. Ask them how their day is going, not out of routine, but out of genuine interest. Say something like, "I was just thinking about you and wanted to hear how your day's been. Is there anything you'd like for dinner tonight?" This simple act of care shows that you're not just thinking about them but are also invested in their well-being and happiness.

Marriage was designed to be a lifelong commitment—a promise to love and cherish each other through the ups and downs. But in difficult moments, it's easy to feel overwhelmed and tempted by advice that encourages giving up. Friends may say things like, "You deserve better," or, "Why stay when it's this hard?" While they may mean well, no one truly understands your relationship except you and your partner.

Instead of leaning on worldly advice, turn to God for guidance. Ask Him to teach you how to love selflessly, how to forgive fully, and how to be the spouse your partner needs. Pray for strength to persevere and wisdom to navigate the challenges you're facing. When you lean on God, you're inviting His peace and understanding into your marriage.

It's natural to feel disheartened when your efforts don't seem to be reciprocated. Maybe your partner won't say much about the note, or they might dismiss your call. But don't let that discourage you. These small acts of love are not wasted; they're planting seeds of kindness and patience that can grow over time.

Love isn't always easy, but it's worth fighting for. Marriage is a journey of learning and growing together, even in the hardest seasons. Trust that your consistent efforts, no matter how small, are building a foundation for healing and reconciliation. Stay focused, stay hopeful, and let today's note and call be another step in the direction of love. You're moving forward, and every step counts.

DAY 8

Start With Effective Communication

Every relationship starts with a spark, a connection that draws you to your partner. Somewhere along the way, life may have dimmed that light. But it's still there, waiting to be rekindled.

Find a quiet moment to talk with your partner. Start by asking gently, "Can we take a little time to talk? I'd love to hear your thoughts about something." Timing matters here. You might bring it up while lying in bed, relaxing on the couch, or even as you're finishing a task. The setting doesn't have to be perfect; the key is your approach—warm, calm, and genuine.

Once you have their attention, guide the conversation with love. Ask them, "Do you remember how we fell in love? What was it about me that first caught your eye?" These questions are not about seeking compliments or reassurance. They are about reconnecting, remembering the foundation of your relationship, and opening a door to intimacy.

As they share, listen carefully. Let their words take you back to the time when your hearts were full of excitement and possibility. Maybe it was the way you laughed, the kindness in your gestures, or a moment when they felt truly seen and understood by you. Let their memories remind you of the love that started it all.

Then, share your side. Be honest and heartfelt. Tell them what made you fall for them—their smile, their confidence, their compassion. Let your words flow naturally, without holding back. This is your opportunity to express your feelings and remind them why they became your person.

These moments of shared vulnerability can be incredibly powerful. They remind you both that beneath the challenges, disagreements, and hurts, there is still a bond worth fighting for. You're not just partners in life's struggles; you're two people who chose each other out of love.

Marriage takes two people to make it work. No magic wand can erase the difficulties or fix the cracks. It requires effort, patience, and a willingness to meet each other halfway. Conversations like this, though seemingly simple, are part of that effort. They create space for understanding, healing, and rebuilding trust.

If your partner seems reluctant, don't take it as a failure. Their walls may still be up, and that's okay. What matters is that you're trying to plant seeds of love and connection with your words and actions. Over time, these seeds can grow into something beautiful.

Relationships thrive when both partners nurture them. By revisiting your love story, you're reminding yourselves of the foundation you built together. It's a step toward reigniting the spark and showing your partner that you're willing to put in the work to keep your marriage alive.

Hold on to these moments and let them guide you forward, one day at a time.

DAY 9

Rebuilding Through Prayer

I want to guide you toward one of the most powerful acts of love you can offer your partner and your marriage: prayer. In the morning and evening, take a moment to kneel, hold hands, and pray together. Sing if you can, even if it's just a simple hymn or a heartfelt song of gratitude and hope. This might feel unfamiliar or even uncomfortable at first, but prayer invites God into your relationship. He is the anchor that steadies the ship in the storm.

When you approach your partner, do so with gentleness and sincerity. Say something like, "Hey love, can we pray together? I feel like we both need God's guidance right now." This is not about forcing them into prayer but about inviting them into a sacred moment of connection—one that strengthens not just your bond with each other, but also with God.

Your partner's response may surprise you. They might agree, hesitant but willing to try. Or, they might say, "No way," pulling the covers over their head or brushing you off. If they reject the invitation, don't let it discourage you. Kneel alone and pray for them, for your marriage, and for the strength to keep moving forward. Let your love and faith guide you, even in the absence of their participation.

Prayer is more than words. It's an act of surrender and humility, a recognition that some battles are too big to fight on our own. When you pray together, you're acknowledging that your marriage isn't just between two people—it's a union under God. By turning to Him, you're saying, We can't do this alone, but with You, we can overcome anything.

Even if your partner doesn't join in right away, they'll notice your efforts. They might wonder, What's going on?

Why are they doing this? At first, they might feel uneasy or even resistant. But over time, the consistency of your prayers will speak louder than any argument or plea. It will show them that you're not giving up on them or your marriage.

Prayer has a unique way of softening hearts and creating space for healing. It reconnects relationships by bringing both partners into the presence of the One who created love itself. Through prayer, you're not just asking for help; you're also opening your heart to forgiveness, patience, and understanding and these are qualities essential for any marriage to thrive.

Remember, God is always ready to help when you call on Him. He sees your struggles, your tears, and your efforts. Even when it feels like nothing is changing, trust that He is working behind the scenes, strengthening you and preparing your marriage for restoration.

DAY 10

Do Something That's Unexpected Of You

Today, you'll do something different and unexpected. Think of a house chore your partner usually handles. It could be doing the dishes, folding the laundry, taking out the trash, or vacuuming the living room. Whatever it is, take it upon yourself to do that task without being asked. It might sound small, but trust me, this simple act can make a big impact.

Picture this: your partner comes home and notices the kitchen is spotless or the laundry is folded neatly. They might stand there for a moment, blinking in disbelief. They might even ask, "Did you do this?" And when you answer with a casual, "Yeah, I thought I'd take care of it," you might just see a flicker of surprise or even appreciation in their eyes.

Why does this work? Because it's unexpected. When you step outside of your usual roles and take on a task your partner doesn't expect, it shows effort. It tells them, I see what you do, and I value it. I want to help ease your load.

But don't stop there. Once the chore is done, find a moment to sit down with your partner and ask, "How was your day?" Now, here's the key—give them your full attention. Put your phone away, mute the TV, and listen. Let them talk without interrupting, judging, or jumping in with solutions. Sometimes, people just need to be heard, and your quiet presence can mean more than any advice you could offer.

If they start venting about something that seems trivial to you, resist the urge to roll your eyes or say, "That's not a big deal." Instead, nod, validate their feelings, and go with the flow. You might even throw in a lighthearted comment like, "Wow, that sounds like a plot twist no one asked for!" to bring a smile to their face. Humor can be a great way to lighten the mood without dismissing their concerns.

You might be wondering, Why should I do this? They don't notice my efforts anyway. Here's the thing: it's not just about them noticing. It's about showing them, in small but consistent ways, that you care. When you make an effort to listen and lighten their load, you're building a foundation of trust and goodwill.

Doing something unexpected keeps things interesting. You might even enjoy the look of surprise on their face when they realize you took care of that chore they've been dreading. Who knows? It might even inspire them to return the favor someday.

Marriage isn't about grand gestures every day. It's about the little things—the unexpected acts of kindness, the willingness to listen, and the effort to make your partner feel valued. So go ahead, tackle that chore, and lend them an ear. It might seem small, but these moments have the power to strengthen your bond in ways you can't yet

Marriage is one of life's most profound commitments. It's the union of two souls, a journey where love, understanding, and patience must grow together. A solid relationship is not built on fleeting emotions or perfect moments but cultivated in the messy, imperfect, and sometimes painful parts of life. It's here, in the midst of challenges, that real love has the chance to thrive.

When you build a strong foundation with your partner, you're creating more than a lasting relationship. You're crafting a safe space where both of you can grow, heal, and dream together. A marriage with a strong bond becomes a shelter in life's storms, a place of comfort when the world feels overwhelming.

To be honest, building this kind of relationship is not easy. It takes effort, intentionality, and a willingness to choose your partner every single day, even when the emotions fade or conflicts arise. Every word spoken, every small action, and every choice you make either strengthens or weakens the connection you share.

Think of it this way: a marriage is like a garden. Neglect it, and weeds of resentment and misunderstanding will overtake it. But tend to it with acts of kindness, communication, and forgiveness and it will bloom beautifully. This doesn't mean perfection; it means persistence. Even when the soil feels dry or the growth seems slow, the care you give will make all the difference.

A solid marriage matters because it affects everything else—your happiness, your family, and even your future. It becomes the legacy you leave behind, a living example of love, resilience, and commitment.
As you embark on this journey to rebuild and strengthen your relationship, remember that no step is too small. Whether it's a kind word, a thoughtful gesture, or a moment of shared prayer, every act of love adds a brick to the foundation of your marriage.

This journey is not about fixing your partner or demanding change. It's about showing up, being present, and committing to the process. Because when you invest in your marriage, you're not just saving a relationship—you're creating something extraordinary, a love that can withstand anything life throws your way.

PART THREE: Physical Intimacy

DAY 11

The Power of a Compliment and a Helping Hand

Today's task is simple yet powerful. You need to give your partner a genuine compliment. Tell them they look great, notice something about their outfit or hairstyle, and say it with sincerity. If they're getting ready for work, offer to adjust their tie, smooth out their shirt, or fix a stray strand of hair. These small acts of care can create a ripple effect in your relationship.

Why does this work? Compliments remind your partner that they are seen, appreciated, and valued. Life gets busy, and sometimes, in the rush of everyday responsibilities, we forget to notice the little things. A kind word or a thoughtful gesture can cut through the noise and remind your partner that they still hold a special place in your heart.

Marriage thrives when both partners feel valued. When you take a moment to appreciate how they look or offer to help with something as small as fixing a collar or tying a shoelace, you're saying more than just, "You look good." You're saying, "I see you. I care about you. You matter to me."

Think back to the early days of your relationship. Do you remember how you used to notice everything about them—the way their smile lit up the room, the way they carried themselves, the little quirks that made them unique? Back then, you probably couldn't stop yourself from complimenting them. And when they returned the favor, it made your heart skip a beat.

But over time, life happens. The compliments fade, replaced by routines, responsibilities, and sometimes, unspoken frustrations. Today is your chance to bring back that spark by focusing on the little things you once cherished.

When you compliment your partner, you're not just boosting their confidence but strengthening your bond. Even if they act shy or brush it off with a joke, deep down, they'll remember that moment. They'll feel a warmth that words can't always express.

And if you want to add a bit of humor, go for it! Say something like, "Wow, you look so good today—are you trying to distract me from my chores?" or "Is it legal to look this amazing before breakfast?" Humour softens the moment, making it feel light and fun while still delivering the message of love.

Marriage is about partnership, and part of that is looking out for each other. It's the small acts like helping fix a button, brushing lint off a jacket, or complimenting a hairstyle that remind your partner you're paying attention. These moments might seem insignificant, but they add up to create a relationship built on care and connection.

So today, notice your partner. Compliment them. Offer to help with something small. These little gestures are the threads that weave a strong and lasting bond. They say, without words, I'm here for you. We're in this together. And that, my friend, is what marriage is all about.

DAY 12

Small Acts of Care that Speak Volumes

Divorce doesn't just break a marriage; it shatters dreams, disrupts families, and leaves scars on hearts that take years to heal.

Now is the time to take a step to rebuild those dreams and mend the connection you once had. Start the day by bringing your partner breakfast in bed. It doesn't have to be a lavish spread but something simple like a cup of coffee, toast, or their favorite morning treat will do. Later in the evening, offer to give them a massage. These acts, though seemingly small, carry immense value.

Why does this work? These gestures are more than just acts of kindness. They show your partner that you're thinking of them and that their comfort and happiness matter to you. In a world where everyone seems to be rushing, pausing to care for your partner in such thoughtful ways communicates love in its purest form.

Bringing breakfast in bed is an intimate and nurturing act. It says, "I want to start your day by taking care of you." It creates a moment of closeness and breaks the monotony of routine mornings. If your partner responds with surprise, a smile, or even skepticism, let it slide. You're not doing this for instant gratitude but planting seeds of affection and rebuilding trust.

Later, as the day winds down, offering a massage can work wonders. It's a physical yet gentle way to reconnect, breaking down walls of tension both emotional and physical. A massage isn't just about easing sore muscles; it's about saying, "I want you to relax. I'm here to support you."

Think back to when you first fell in love. You probably found joy in caring for each other, in doing thoughtful things just to see them smile. Over time, life's challenges may have dulled those moments, but they don't have to disappear. Acts of care like these remind your partner and yourself of the love that brought you together.

Divorce often happens when couples stop seeing and valuing each other. These small acts are ways to say, "I still see you, and I still care." They help to soften hearts that may have grown cold and remind both of you of the beauty of partnership.

Even if your partner doesn't respond the way you hope, don't give up. Building a bridge takes time and persistence. You're not just trying to win them over but showing them what love looks like when it's patient and selfless.

So, start the day with breakfast in bed. End it with a gentle massage. And in between, carry the mindset of love and service. These small acts may seem insignificant, but their impact is profound. They say I'm here, I care, and I choose us. And that choice can make all the difference.

DAY 13

Sing, Dance, and Rekindle the Magic

Music has a way of breaking down walls, evoking memories, and speaking straight to the heart. Today, you'll use the magic of melody to reconnect with your partner in a playful, meaningful way. Start by picking a song that reminds you of your partner. Maybe it's the song you danced to at your wedding, a tune that played during one of your dates, or a favorite you both sing along to in the car. If nothing comes to mind, choose something romantic and heartfelt. Then, sing it to them maybe karaoke style.

Yes, sing! Don't worry about hitting the perfect notes. The beauty lies in the effort, the joy, and the connection it creates. Watching you sing to them will catch your partner off guard in the best way, making them smile, laugh, or even tear up. They'll feel noticed, appreciated, and loved. Once your performance is over and they're still smiling or laughing (trust me, they will), take it a step further. Play a slow, romantic song, stretch out your hand, and invite them to dance. If they hesitate, don't let that stop you. Tease them playfully, tug their arm gently, or give them that mischievous look that says, "You're not getting out of this!"

And if they're being extra stubborn, which could be possible, take a bold step and drag them off the couch or chair with a laugh, wrap your arms around their waist, and guide them into the rhythm of the song. Place a soft kiss on their forehead or cheek, touch their chest lightly, and let the music do the talking.

While you're swaying together, let your words flow from the heart. Whisper something sweet, like, "You still make my heart skip a beat," or "Dancing with you feels like coming home." Speak your love, even if it feels awkward at first. Vulnerability is the bridge to a deeper connection, and your partner will feel your sincerity.

Now, not every partner will jump up eagerly to dance or gush over the gesture. Some may hesitate, joke their way out of it, or even pull back. If that happens, don't be discouraged. Smile, hold your ground, and remember: this isn't about instant results. It's about showing consistent love, even when it's not immediately reciprocated.

And don't forget to laugh at yourself! If your singing was a little off-key or your dance moves were clumsy, embrace it. Humour keeps the mood light and shows your partner you're not taking yourself too seriously. You're creating a memory, not auditioning for a talent show.

If, by chance, your partner doesn't give in today, that's okay because you still got Day 14 and beyond. What matters most is your effort, your persistence, and your commitment to reigniting the spark in your relationship. Love isn't about grand gestures; it's about the simple, heartfelt moments that remind your partner they are cherished.

So, sing your heart out, dance like no one's watching, and let love lead the way. One step at a time, you're rebuilding something truly beautiful.

DAY 14

You Are Not Too Old To Play Games

Love isn't just about grand gestures or candlelit dinners. Love also involves laughter, fun, and reconnecting with that playful spark that brought you two together in the first place. Relationships can often feel weighed down by responsibilities, but today, we're going to shake things up. It's time to reignite the flame in a way that's lighthearted and fun.

Here's the plan: play a video game together or revisit an activity you both loved during your dating days or early marriage. Think about those carefree moments when you were laughing until your sides hurt, teasing each other, and feeling so in sync. It could be anything—a board game, cards, karaoke, or even a silly DIY project. If video games are your thing, pick a fun and interactive one that's easy to enjoy together.

And if you have kids, invite them to join the fun! Transform it into a family gathering that's filled with joy, laughter, and connection. Nothing warms the heart more than seeing everyone you love coming together, sharing smiles, and creating new memories.

Now, during the activity, slip in some random questions to keep things interesting. Ask your partner things like, "What's one thing you loved most about our first date?" or "If we could relive one moment from our past, what would it be?" These questions aren't just icebreakers but they're tiny windows into your shared history and a gentle nudge to bring back those cherished memories.

So, why does this work? Play is an incredible way to break down barriers. It dissolves tension, replaces formality with spontaneity, and reminds you both of the joy in each other's company. When you're laughing, strategizing, or competing (good-naturedly, of course), the walls of resentment or silence begin to crumble.

And if your partner is hesitant, don't force it. Start playing anyway, your enthusiasm might just be contagious. Show them that you're willing to put in the effort, even if it means laughing at yourself or messing up during the game. Humour is an amazing icebreaker, and seeing you let loose might encourage them to join in.

If you have kids, this is a beautiful opportunity to show them what love looks like—playful, forgiving, and being intentional. It sends the message that marriage isn't just about serious moments but also about enjoying each other's company, even after years together.

By the end of this day, you'll find that playing together can rekindle more than just laughter. It brings back those tender feelings from when love was fresh and life felt simple. And if your partner doesn't completely open up today, don't worry. You've planted a seed. Every step you take is a step closer to rediscovering the magic that's always been there.

So, grab the controllers, shuffle the cards, or roll the dice. Let play be your love language today, and watch as the joy spreads like wildfire. Because love, when nurtured with laughter, is truly unstoppable.

DAY 15

Strengthen Your Bond Through Shared Experiences

Sometimes, the best way to reconnect with your partner is by stepping outside your bubble and sharing experiences with other couples. Today, your mission is to plan an outing or activity with other couples—friends you trust, respect, and feel comfortable around. This isn't just about socializing; it's about rediscovering your relationship in a fresh and engaging environment.

Whether it's a cozy dinner, a relaxing beach hangout, a visit to an open market, or even a fun ice cream date, the goal is to enjoy a shared experience. Surrounding yourself with other couples can create a positive atmosphere that inspires and uplifts your relationship. It gives you and your partner a chance to see each other through the eyes of others, sparking appreciation and even a little bit of pride.

Why does this work so well? First, it adds variety. Doing something different and involving others can shake up your routine, giving you both something to look forward to and reminisce about later. Second, it subtly reminds you of the joy of partnership. As you watch other couples interact, you may find yourself reflecting on the good moments in your relationship.

During this outing, try to engage in lighthearted conversation with your partner and the group. Bring up funny memories or moments you've shared. If the setting feels right, ask your partner playful or meaningful questions, like, "What's one thing we haven't done in a while that you miss?" or "If you could plan our dream date, what would it be?"

Being around other couples also helps foster a sense of community. It's easy to feel isolated when a marriage is struggling, but seeing others navigate their relationships can remind you that every couple has their ups and downs.

You're not alone in this journey, and there's strength in shared experiences.

Now, here's a gentle reminder: this outing isn't about comparing your relationship to anyone else's. It's about celebrating what makes your bond unique while learning from the love and laughter around you. If your partner seems distant or uninterested during the outing, don't take it to heart. Focus on the positive moments, no matter how small, and trust that even the simplest gestures are planting seeds of healing and reconnection.

By the end of this day, you may notice a shift in how you see each other. It could be in the way they smile at you across the table or the warmth in their tone as you talk. These moments, though subtle, are signs of rebuilding. Love grows in shared joy, and today is all about creating memories that remind you both of why you chose each other in the first place. So, plan that outing, laugh freely, and let the power of connection work its magic.

Sometimes, the company of others is exactly what you need to bring the two of you closer together.

PART FOUR: Building Emotional Bridges

DAY 16

Kill The Parasite That's Poisoning Your Love

Every relationship faces challenges, but some challenges don't come from the outside but they come from within. Today is about facing yourself and asking the hard question: What am I holding onto that's destroying my marriage?

A parasite doesn't just weaken you, it sucks the life out of your bond. Whether it's an addiction to drinking, smoking, pornography, flirting, or any other unhealthy habit, these behaviors are at the foundation of your relationship. Maybe your partner has begged you to stop for years. Maybe they've cried, yelled, or withdrawn because they feel unheard and unloved. And yet, the cycle continues.

Today, it's time to stop. Not tomorrow. Not when the time is right. Right now. Because every moment you let these habits linger, you're choosing them over your partner, your love, and your future together.

Think about it: trust is the heartbeat of a relationship, and these habits are like daggers stabbing at it. When you prioritize a harmful addiction over your spouse, it sends a message, even if unintentional: You are not enough for me. No matter how much you try to cover it up, these actions create a wall between you and the person you vowed to cherish.

Take pornography, for instance. It rewires the brain, making real intimacy seem dull in comparison to artificial fantasies. Drinking or smoking may lead to moments of anger, recklessness, or neglect, leaving your partner feeling unprotected and unsafe. Flirting with others is often seen as harmless fun and this is wrong. It's a betrayal that plants seeds of insecurity and doubt in your partner's heart.

But here's the truth: these habits don't define you. You are not your mistakes. You are not your past. You have the power to choose love over addiction, faithfulness over temptation, and healing over destruction.

Let today be the day you start killing the parasite. Begin by acknowledging it. Don't deny its existence or justify it with excuses. Be honest with yourself and, if possible, with your partner. Say, "I know this habit is hurting us, and I don't want to let it control me anymore."

Seek support if you need it. Breaking free from addiction isn't easy, but it's worth every ounce of effort. Pray for strength. Seek counseling or join a support group. Whatever it takes, fight for your marriage with everything you've got.

Always remember that love isn't just about saying I love you but showing it through action. By choosing to let go of these harmful habits, you're telling your partner,

DAY 17

Love in the Kitchen

Love isn't just spoken but it's lived, shared, and expressed in the small, unexpected moments of everyday life. Today, let those moments unfold in the heart of your home: the kitchen. Start with three simple but powerful words: I love you. Say them when your partner least expects it, maybe while they're reading, watching TV, or even scrolling through their phone. It may catch them off guard, but it's a beautiful way to remind them of your feelings.

Now, here's where things get exciting: invite your partner to join you in the kitchen. Tell them you've discovered a new recipe and would love to make it together. There's something magical about creating a meal side by side, blending flavors while sharing laughs, stories, and even playful banter. It's not just about cooking; it's about bonding.

Cooking together is an intimate experience. It's a space where you can collaborate, support one another, and even make a little mess together. But here's an important tip: don't let the mess or mistakes ruin the moment. If your partner accidentally spills something or burns a piece of toast, laugh it off. Say something lighthearted like, "Looks like we just invented a new twist to this recipe!" Scolding, nagging, or complaining will only add tension. The goal is connection, not perfection.

As you cook, set the mood. Play some soft music in the background or choose a playlist you both enjoy. Wear something that makes you feel confident and attractive. This isn't about being flashy—it's about reminding your partner of the spark that drew them to you. If you've got a favorite fitted shirt, stylish apron, or those form-fitting jeans that show off your best features, now's the time to pull them out. Let your attire speak a silent message: I want to look good for you.

The kitchen can be a space of shared laughter and love. Sneak in a compliment while chopping vegetables or stir-frying: "You're so good at this and I think we make a great team." Or, if the moment feels right, steal a quick kiss while they're distracted. These little gestures may seem small, but they leave a lasting impression.

When the meal is finally ready, sit down together and enjoy the fruits of your teamwork. Raise a glass to celebrate the simple yet meaningful experience you've just shared. And if your partner isn't a fan of cooking or declines your invitation, don't let it dampen your spirit. Cook the meal with love and present it to them with a smile.

A kitchen isn't just a place where meals are made; it's where bonds are strengthened. Today, let the chopping, stirring, and seasoning become metaphors for the effort and care you're putting into your marriage. It's a reminder that love isn't just about the grand gestures but sharing life's simple moments, even if it's over a simmering pot of soup. Let this day be a flavorful step toward reconciling the love you both deserve.

DAY 18

Step Outside To Step Closer

A broken marriage doesn't have to remain broken, and a lost connection doesn't have to stay lost. Love is a living thing; it may fade, but it can also be rekindled. Today's challenge is about stepping out both physically and emotionally. Plan something outdoors with your partner. It could be a scenic road trip, a peaceful road walk, or a fun photo walk to capture the beauty around you and in each other.

Sometimes, the walls of our home carry the weight of unresolved arguments, hurt feelings, or silence. Stepping outside gives you both a chance to leave that heaviness behind, even if just for a while. Fresh air, new surroundings, and shared experiences have a way of bringing clarity and opening the door for reconnection.

When suggesting this outing, make it casual yet thoughtful. Say something like, "I've been thinking we haven't had a proper day out together in a while. How about we take a drive and explore somewhere new?" Or, if time is limited, suggest a short walk around your neighborhood or a local park. For those who enjoy taking pictures, a photo walk could be a fun way to capture moments and relive the joy of simply being together.

Why does this matter? Because intimacy isn't just about physical closeness or romantic gestures. It's also about sharing meaningful moments, creating memories, and showing your partner that they matter. These little gestures like holding hands during a walk or stopping to buy them their favorite snack along the way are quiet yet powerful ways to communicate love.

Healing a broken bond takes intentionality. It's not about who was right or wrong; it's about finding ways to meet in the middle again. An outdoor activity might seem simple, but it can spark conversations that have been left unsaid for too long. Maybe your partner will open up about something weighing on their heart. Maybe you'll both laugh over an old memory or discover something new about each other.

If your partner resists the idea at first, don't push. Offer to go on your own but leave the invitation open. Sometimes, curiosity or the realization that they might miss out will draw them in. And even if they don't join, use the time to reflect on how you can continue building the bridge between you.

As you're out together, remind yourself that every broken marriage can be fixed if both people are willing to try. It won't happen overnight, but each small step counts. Love is resilient, it can withstand storms, and with care, it can grow even stronger.

This isn't just about spending time together; it's about showing your partner that you're willing to make the effort, that you still value the relationship, and that you're committed to healing what's been hurt. Step outside and step closer, one small yet meaningful moment at a time.

DAY 19

A Romantic Intimate Night

Intimacy is the language of love that words often fail to speak. It's a bridge that reconnects two hearts, reminding them of what they once shared and the passion that brought them together. Today, it's time to embrace that connection not just as a physical act but as a deeper way to express love, vulnerability, and trust.

This time, you're not just going through the motions. You're reigniting a flame that may have dimmed over time. Prepare yourself with intention and care. Choose an outfit that makes you feel confident and irresistible, something your partner won't be able to look away from. Whether it's elegant lingerie, a well-fitted outfit, or simply the way you carry yourself, let your appearance radiate desire and love.

Approach your spouse gently. Warm kisses on their forehead, a soft touch on their hand, or playful caresses can break the invisible walls that may have built up between you. Whisper something heartfelt, like, "I've missed being this close to you," or simply let your actions do the talking. Pay attention to the little things—running your fingers through their hair, tracing your hands along their shoulders, just anything that makes them feel cherished and desired.

Why is this important? Because intimacy is about more than physical closeness. It's about emotional vulnerability, a moment where you both let your guard down and connect on the deepest level. For a partner who may have felt neglected, this act can be a healing balm, a way of saying without words, "You still mean everything to me."

If your partner is hesitant or unsure, take your time. This isn't about rushing; it's about creating a space where they feel safe and loved. Let your gestures speak volumes—your patience, your tenderness, and your genuine desire to reconnect. Maybe they've missed this closeness but didn't know how to reach out. Maybe they've felt distant and are longing to feel wanted again.

Intimacy, when given freely and lovingly, has the power to mend even the deepest wounds. It can remind you both of the love that started it all, the connection that's worth fighting for.

This isn't just about the physical act of being together; it's about reigniting a sense of belonging. It's about reminding your partner that no matter how far apart you've felt, there's always a way back to each other. At this moment, let love take center stage and watch how the walls begin to crumble, making way for a stronger, more united bond.

DAY 20

Winning The War In Your Mind

Today, the challenge takes a slightly different turn. It's not a day off, but it's a day for introspection, a time to step back and look at the bigger picture of your relationship. You've been actively pouring love, effort, and care into your marriage over the past few days, but now it's time to turn inward and reflect.

Take a quiet moment for yourself, away from the noise and distractions. Find an article or a story about marriage, divorce, or reconciliation, find something that resonates with your journey. Read it with an open heart. Let it remind you of the stakes and the possibilities, of the fragile yet powerful beauty of love and connection.

Now, close your eyes and think back to the beginning of your relationship. Picture the first time you met your partner, the laughter you shared, and the dreams you built together. Remember the little things that made your heart flutter: the way they smiled, the sound of their voice, or the way they made you feel seen and loved. Those memories aren't just fleeting snapshots—they're the foundation of what you've built together.

Ask yourself these questions

What has changed since those early days?

Is the love still there, hidden beneath the hurts and misunderstandings?

Could this relationship still flourish if given the right care and attention?

Then, let yourself imagine a life without your partner. Not just the initial relief you might feel if the pain were to end, but the reality of starting over. Would your world be truly better without them? Could anyone else understand you the way they do or at least did once? Perhaps you'd meet someone kinder, or perhaps someone worse. But here's the truth: every person comes with their flaws, just as you do. No one is perfect. The key to a successful relationship is learning to embrace those imperfections with love, patience, and understanding.

If there's even the smallest part of you that wants to fight for this relationship, hold on to it. That flicker of hope is a sign that something is worth saving. Love isn't always easy, and it doesn't thrive on grand gestures alone. It's built on the everyday choices to forgive, to stay, and to try again, even when it feels like the easiest option is to walk away.

Think of your partner's flaws. Have they been difficult? Sure. But ask yourself: Have you been difficult too? Relationships aren't about perfection; they're about learning to love through imperfections. It's about creating a space where growth, healing, and reconciliation can happen.

Take today to center yourself and reconnect with your intentions. Reflect on the journey so far and the road ahead. This isn't just about saving your marriage but saving the part of you that believed in love, commitment, and forever.

If your heart still carries even a whisper of desire to rebuild this relationship, don't ignore it. That whisper is where healing begins. Love, after all, isn't just something that happens to us. It's a choice we make every day. And today, you have the chance to choose it again.

PART FIVE: Creating Lasting Memories

DAY 21

Reconnecting Through the Little Things

Today is about rekindling intimacy in the simplest, most meaningful way which is sharing a bath or shower. It might feel like a small gesture, but it has the power to rebuild a bond that's been weakened by the weight of time and misunderstandings.

When you see your partner preparing for a shower, surprise them by stepping in with a playful smile and a warm heart. Let this shared moment be a quiet escape from the world, a time to focus only on each other. Wash away the stress, the hurt, and even the walls that may have grown between you. Let the water symbolize a fresh start, cleansing the wounds of the past and opening a door to a more connected future.

Couples often think that saving a marriage requires grand gestures, but the truth is that love thrives in the little things. Holding hands under the stream of water, helping each other lather shampoo, or even exchanging light-hearted jokes can spark feelings you thought were long gone. These small, tender moments remind you of the joy of simply being close to one another.

If trust has been broken, if you've caught your partner cheating or suspect they've sought attention elsewhere, this can be a hard step to take. But let's reflect on the "why." Sometimes, infidelity isn't about love or attraction but a desperate search for something missing. That doesn't make it right, but it highlights how vital care, attention, and affection are in a marriage.

This shower isn't just about physical closeness; it's a gesture of emotional vulnerability. By stepping into this intimate moment, you're showing your partner that you still care, that you're willing to forgive, and that you believe in rebuilding what was broken.

The truth is, nobody else will ever truly understand your partner the way you do. That connection, built over years of shared laughter, tears, and dreams, is not something that can be easily replaced. If you let love guide your actions, even in the face of betrayal, you might find that the bond you rebuild is stronger than ever.

So, take this opportunity to reconnect in a way that words can't achieve. Let the warmth of your touch and the simplicity of your presence say what your heart feels. Marriage isn't about perfection or never making mistakes, marriage means committing to grow, forgive, and love one another through it all.

And if your partner resists or pulls away, don't lose hope. These gestures are steps, not magic solutions. Trust the process, and remember that every effort you make is an investment in your love and your future.

DAY 22

Let Love Speak Through Stories

This task is simple yet deeply impactful. Listen to a podcast with your partner. Not just any podcast, but one that speaks to the heart of what matters: love, trust, and the delicate threads that hold a marriage together. A good podcast can open doors to understanding in ways that regular conversation sometimes cannot. It's like letting someone else articulate the emotions, struggles, and solutions you've been trying to express.

Find a podcast episode about the realities of marriage—the beauty, the challenges, and how love and trust can be rebuilt even after painful moments. Topics like how divorce affects families and children or ways to reconnect when love feels distant can resonate deeply.

Timing is everything. Wait until your partner is around, maybe during a quiet evening or while you're both relaxing at home. With a gentle smile, say, "I found something I thought we might listen to together. It's about love and relationships and I think we might learn something." Don't push; just play the podcast and let the words work their magic.

If your partner resists or claims they're not interested, don't let that deter you. Simply start playing it in the background. They may not sit next to you, but they will hear the words. Let the podcast do the talking. The stories and advice will seep in, planting seeds of thought and reflection. Sometimes, it's easier for people to absorb truths when they come from someone else, especially in a non-confrontational setting.

Podcasts have a way of making people feel seen and understood. Hearing others share similar struggles, triumphs, and practical advice can inspire a sense of hope and possibility. It can gently remind both of you that you're not alone in your challenges and that there are proven ways to rebuild love and trust.

Marriage is a journey, and just like any road trip, it sometimes requires stopping to refuel and check the map. A podcast like this can serve as that refuel—a moment to reflect, learn, and recalibrate.

Even if your partner doesn't openly engage, remember that every small step counts. Listening together isn't just about the words; it's about creating an opportunity for connection. It shows your partner that you care enough to try, to learn, and to grow.

Trust that these moments, no matter how small they seem, are building blocks toward something greater. Keep showing up, keep trying, and let love do the rest.

DAY 23

The Power of Deep Conversations

Today is about peeling back the layers of your relationship and getting to the heart of your connection. It's not just about fixing what's broken; it's about understanding each other in ways you may have forgotten. Life's chaos often overshadows the simple beauty of sitting with your partner and asking, "What's on your mind? What are your fears, your dreams, your hopes?"

Find a quiet moment when the two of you can sit together without distractions. It could be in the living room, at the kitchen table, or even outside under the stars. Start the conversation gently: "I want to know more about you—your fears, your strengths, your weaknesses. Even if I thought I knew, I want to hear it all again, directly from you."

This isn't just a question; it's an invitation. An invitation to vulnerability, to trust, and to let walls crumble. Be prepared to listen, truly listen, without interrupting or judging. If your spouse hesitates or brushes it off with a laugh, stay patient. Let them know you're not rushing, this moment is theirs.

As the conversation flows, open your heart too. Share your dreams and fears. Tell them specific things you love about them. Don't settle for vague compliments but be precise. Instead of saying, "I love you because you're kind," try, "I love how you go out of your way to make sure everyone around you feels seen and valued." These little details show how closely you observe and cherish them.

Talk about your shared vision for the future. Where do you see yourselves in five or ten years? What kind of life do you want to create together? Discuss your family, your children, and the values you want to instill in them. Let this conversation remind you both of the reasons you chose each other in the first place and the potential that still exists for your relationship.

This moment isn't about fixing everything in one sitting. It's about opening a door to empathy, understanding, and a renewed connection. Often, marriages break down not because of big arguments but because of small, everyday disconnects. Conversations like this help rebuild the bridge.

Remember, vulnerability is the heart of intimacy. When you share your inner world with someone, it fosters a deep sense of closeness. This is your opportunity to let your partner know you're not giving up, that you still see them, love them, and want to walk through life together.

The beauty of this moment is that it plants seeds for tomorrow. Even if the conversation feels heavy or awkward at first, trust that it's working. Slowly, it's knitting back the threads of love and trust that may have frayed over time.

Day 24

Seeking Help Together

There comes a point when love alone may not be enough to bridge the gaps that have formed between you and your spouse. That's okay. Love isn't about having all the answers; it's about knowing when to ask for help. Today is the day you take a brave step forward by suggesting professional guidance.

In a calm and heartfelt moment, sit with your partner and say, "I've been thinking about us, and I believe we owe it to each other to try everything we can to make this work. I've reached out to a marriage counselor and scheduled an appointment for the day after tomorrow. It would mean so much to me if we could do this together."

If they respond positively, hold their hand and thank them. Let them know how much it means to you that they're willing to take this step. Assure them that this isn't about pointing fingers or assigning blame. It's about creating a safe space where both of you can be heard and supported.

But what if they hesitate? What if they refuse? This is where you must summon every ounce of patience and understanding. Don't argue or try to coerce them. Instead, ask gently, "Can you help me understand why you feel this way? I truly want to know what's hurting you so much that you feel like you can't take this step with me."

This question isn't just about getting an answer; it's about showing them you're listening and that their feelings matter. Your partner might not open up immediately, especially if they've been carrying years of pain or resentment. But your calm persistence and genuine concern might plant a seed of reflection in their heart.

If emotions start to rise, don't hold back your vulnerability. Let them see how much this means to you.

Say, "I need your support for this, just this once. I can't do this alone anymore. You're important to me, and I want us to heal together. Please, let's try."

Sometimes, people resist because they fear judgment or feel they've failed. Reassure your partner that seeking help isn't a sign of failure but it's a sign of strength. It's a testament to how much you both value what you've built together.

And if, at the end of the conversation, they still refuse? Don't give up. Keep the appointment for yourself. Attend the session, listen to the counselor's advice, and use the tools you gain to continue fostering change at home. Your willingness to keep trying, even when things seem one-sided, speaks volumes about your commitment.

Marriage is a partnership, but sometimes one person has to take the lead in difficult moments. Be that person today. Lead with love, humility, and hope. And remember, every step forward, no matter how small, is still progress.

DAY 25

Fulfilling Their Request

Today's focus is on your spouse's desires, the little things they've asked of you that might have slipped through the cracks of daily life. Perhaps they once asked you to make their favorite meal, wear something special for a date, or even try something new in the bedroom. These requests, no matter how trivial or bold they seemed at the time, are windows into their heart and the connection they long for with you.

Think back to those moments. What was the one thing they asked for, perhaps weeks or even months ago, that you brushed off or forgot? Maybe it sounded unimportant at the time, or life simply got in the way. But to them, it mattered.

Today, it's your turn to show them that their voice matters. If they want a special dinner, take the time to cook it or order it in. If they asked for a fun, bold outfit for a night out, get dressed with intention, knowing it'll light up their eyes. If they asked for more intimacy or to spice things up, let go of your reservations and meet them where their needs are.

Why is this so important? Because at its core, love is about listening and responding. When we act on the things our partner has shared with us, it sends a powerful message: I hear you. I value you. I want to make you happy.

Now, ask yourself, how would you feel if the roles were reversed? What if your spouse remembered a small request you made long ago and fulfilled it without being reminded? Wouldn't it touch your heart to know that they care enough to act on your desires? That's the gift you're giving today: the joy of being seen, heard, and cherished.

This exercise isn't just about ticking off a request; it's about deepening the bond between you. When you honor your partner's wishes, you're reinforcing trust and showing that their happiness matters to you.

If fulfilling their request requires stepping out of your comfort zone, do it with an open heart. Vulnerability is where true connection begins. And if they ask you why you're suddenly doing this, smile and say, "Because it matters to you, and you matter to me."

Marriage is built on countless small moments where we choose to put our partner first, not out of obligation, but out of love. Today is one of those moments. Whatever it is they've asked for, give it your best. Your effort will speak volumes, and it might just reignite a spark that felt lost.

Love isn't about grand gestures every day. Sometimes, it's simply about saying yes to what your partner wants and watching how that one act of kindness breathes new life into your relationship.

PART SIX: New Experience

DAY 26

The Marriage Therapist

A brave step must be taken together by meeting with a marriage counselor. This isn't just another activity in your journey; it's a chance to truly open your hearts and bridge the gaps that once seemed impossible to close.

As you walk into the counselor's office, be ready to lay everything on the table. This is not about pointing fingers or blaming one another but understanding, healing, and finding a way forward. Marriage counseling is a sacred space, a neutral ground where both of you can voice your emotions without fear of judgment.

When the session begins, hold your partner's hand. It might feel awkward at first, but trust me, it sends a powerful message. In that touch, you're saying, I'm here with you. I'm not giving up on us. Whether they grip your hand tightly or hesitate, their reaction will speak volumes.

They may think to themselves, This marriage truly is till my last breath or even, Why didn't I see this side of my spouse before?

If the counselor asks if you still want a divorce, take a deep breath and remember your vows: for better or worse, till death do us part. Speak those words aloud if you feel it in your heart. Let your spouse hear the weight of the promises you made to each other on that beautiful day when you first said "I do."

Be honest during the session. Share your fears, your pain, and your hopes. Don't hold back about what hurt you in the past, but approach it with grace. Say something like, "These things hurt me deeply, but I see how things are changing, and I want to believe in us again." This is not about reopening old wounds but about clearing the air and letting your partner see why you once felt like walking away—and why you're choosing to stay now.

Marriage counseling is not about fixing blame; it's about fixing the bond. It's about understanding what went wrong and finding tools to rebuild together. It's about hearing each other in ways you may not have before.

This moment is an opportunity to reset your relationship. When you answer the therapist's questions, do so with a genuine heart. Let your partner know that their efforts to change, to heal, and to meet you halfway have not gone unnoticed. And as you sit side by side, hold onto the hope that brought you here in the first place, the belief that love is worth fighting for.

Your journey doesn't end here; it begins anew. Today's step is about learning how to move forward together, as partners who see each other clearly and love each other deeply. Trust in this process, and trust in the power of love to heal even the deepest wounds.

DAY 27

A special Day for You

After weeks of pouring your heart and energy into healing your marriage, today is your day to breathe. You've worked hard to show love, understanding, and care to your partner. Now, it's time to take care of yourself.

This doesn't mean you're giving up on your efforts or taking a step back. It means you're recharging your emotional and mental strength. Relationships thrive when both partners are whole, and today is about nurturing your well-being.

Start the day with something simple and refreshing. Maybe it's a cup of tea or a cold drink that makes you feel at ease. Eat something nourishing, choose foods that energize and comfort you. Don't rush through meals; savor them.

Take a nap if you feel tired. Let your body rest. Or turn on a show or series you enjoy. Laugh at a comedy, immerse yourself in a drama, or indulge in something lighthearted. Whatever you choose, do it for you. Resist the urge to invite your partner to join you. Let them notice your calm and wonder about this new version of you—the one who has been so attentive and caring these past weeks.

This day off is more than just about rest. It's about sending a subtle message to your partner: I'm whole on my own, but I choose to love you. When you take a step back, it gives them a chance to reflect on everything you've been doing. They'll notice the change in the atmosphere of your home, the gentleness you've brought, and the care you've shown.

Let them sit with their thoughts. Let them feel your presence, even in your quietness. This isn't the time to argue, feel sad, or stir up past wounds. It's about balance, showing that while you are deeply committed to your relationship, you also respect yourself enough to take a moment to recharge.

Taking this day for yourself is not selfish; it's necessary. A healthy relationship requires two emotionally balanced people. You've been giving so much love to your partner, and now you need to replenish your well. Self-care is not a luxury; it's a foundation.

As the day winds down, reflect on your journey so far. Think about how far you've come since Day 1. You've faced challenges, opened up your heart, and made intentional choices to build your marriage. Rest in the knowledge that you're doing everything you can to create a better future.

Your partner will notice your calm energy today. They may even ask, "What's on your mind?" or "Why are you so relaxed?" Smile and let them wonder. This quiet strength will leave a lasting impression. Remember, this journey is about love not just for your partner, but also for yourself.

DAY 28

Outdoor Experiences

Today is all about you, celebrating your strength, grace, and individuality. This isn't just another day in the 30 -day challenge; it's a reminder that taking care of yourself is just as important as nurturing your relationship. Self-love and confidence radiate outward, strengthening the love you share with your partner.

Dress to impress not just for anyone else, but for yourself. Choose an outfit that highlights your confidence and makes you feel breathtaking. Let your partner see you as you get ready. If they ask where you're going, respond sweetly and confidently, "I'm meeting a friend for lunch," or "I'm taking the kids out for some fun." Keep your tone light and cheerful. If they offer to tag along or drop you off, let them because it's a sign they're drawn to the energy you're radiating.

If you're a parent, take the kids on an adventure without your partner. This can be a simple outing like going to the park, grabbing ice cream, or a quick shopping trip. If you don't have kids or want some alone time, plan a lunch or dinner date with a close friend, sibling, or even just yourself. Go to a place that brings you joy—a favorite cafe, a cozy restaurant, or a quiet park where you can soak at the moment.

While you're out, enjoy yourself fully. Laugh, relax, and let go of any tension. This is your time to recharge and reconnect with your own identity outside of being a spouse or parent. Think about what makes you happy, your passions, and how far you've come on this journey.

When it's time to head home, don't go empty-handed. Pick up something thoughtful for your spouse—a favorite snack, a flower, or a small gift they'd appreciate. This gesture isn't about extravagance; it's about showing them that even while taking time for yourself, they are still in your thoughts.

As you walk back through the door, let them see the smile on your face. Hand them the gift with a simple, heartfelt comment: "I saw this and thought of you." It's a small yet powerful moment that reminds them of the connection you share.

By taking this time for yourself, you're also demonstrating something beautiful, that you're committed to growing, not just as a couple, but as an individual. This energy is magnetic. It shows your partner that you value yourself and that your love comes from a place of wholeness, not dependency.

Self-care doesn't mean stepping away from love; it means fueling yourself so you can give even more. Today, let your partner see the incredible person they fell in love with—confident, radiant, and full of life. Sometimes, the best way to nurture your marriage is by nurturing yourself.

DAY 29

Sending A Message From The Depth Of Your Heart

You will take a step that requires vulnerability and courage to write a letter to your spouse. This is more than words on paper; it's a piece of your heart, an acknowledgement of your past mistakes, and a promise to do better. Sometimes, the most profound way to mend a relationship is to express genuine regret and a desire to start anew.

Find a quiet moment to reflect on your journey so far. Think about the times you've fallen short whether it was being selfish, impatient, or failing to understand your partner's needs. Let those moments guide your words, but don't let guilt overwhelm you. This letter is not about drowning in self-blame; it's about showing that you see where you went wrong and are willing to change.

Start your letter with sincerity. Write from your heart, not from a place of obligation. Perhaps you could begin with something like, "I've been thinking about us a lot lately, and I realize there are things I should have done differently." Be specific about your mistakes, but avoid being overly harsh on yourself. Share how you feel about the current state of your relationship and your deep desire to rekindle the love that feels absent.

End your letter with a powerful reminder of your commitment: "I love you." These three words, when written from the depths of your soul, have the power to heal and restore.

Now, decide how to deliver this letter. If your spouse is leaving for work, slip it into their bag or hand it to them as they head out. If it's evening, place it on their dinner tray or beside their pillow before bedtime. If you feel more comfortable sending it as a text, that's fine too but try to keep it personal and heartfelt.

Once you've given them the letter, step back. Don't hover or ask if they've read it. Let them take their time to absorb your words. This isn't about seeking immediate validation; it's about creating space for understanding and healing.

By writing this letter, you're showing your spouse that you care deeply about their feelings and are committed to growing together. Words have the power to rebuild trust and reawaken love, especially when they come from a genuine place. Today, let your pen speak the truth of your heart. You may be surprised by the bridges it builds.

DAY 30

The Bold Step Of Hope And Faith

Congratulations! You've reached the final day of this 30-day challenge, designed to heal, rebuild, and reignite the love in your marriage. Today is not about lavish expressions or big conversations. It's about resting, reflecting, and allowing your spouse to take notice.

Stay in bed today. Tuck yourself under the blanket, close your eyes, and let your partner wonder. You're not lying; you're emotionally, mentally, and physically tired. Skip breakfast, leave lunch unattended, and simply rest. This isn't laziness; it's a quiet pause to reflect on how far you've come.

Your spouse will notice. Maybe they'll come into the room, concern written across their face. They might touch your forehead, hold your hand, or ask, "Are you okay?"

Maybe they'll place a soft kiss on your lips or sit beside you in silence, wondering what's wrong. Whatever they do, let them. Let them take the lead for once, even if it's just a small gesture of care.

And if they don't check in, don't let bitterness creep in. And if they finally do, muster all the love you've cultivated over these 30 days, look into their eyes, and say softly, "I love you so much. I'm grateful to God for bringing you into my life." Be sincere. Let your words carry the depth of your heart.

This moment, as simple as it may seem, is powerful. It's a quiet culmination of everything you've done over the past month—every effort, every gesture, every act of love. You've shown your partner that marriage isn't about perfection; it's about persistence, patience, and a willingness to fight for each other.

If, after all of this, your partner still hasn't changed, if they remain distant or unmoved, then take solace in knowing you gave your all. You've done everything in your power to rebuild what was broken. Sometimes, despite our best efforts, people are unwilling or unable to meet us halfway. But this isn't a failure. This is courage.

You can move forward knowing you tried your best, and that's something to be proud of. Whether your marriage finds new life or you decide to walk separate paths, this challenge has taught you the value of love, forgiveness, and intentionality.

The journey doesn't end here. Keep showing love, keep growing, and keep believing in the power of connection. And whatever happens next, know you've done something extraordinary, you fought for love, and that's always worth it.

Conclusion

The pillars of a healthy relationship are not defined by perfection but by intention and the continuous effort to nurture love, build trust, and understand one another. At its core, marriage is a union of two imperfect people who choose each other every single day, despite the challenges. Trust, understanding, and affection are the foundations that uphold this union, and their importance cannot be overstated.

Trust is the heartbeat of any marriage. Without it, every interaction becomes laced with doubt, suspicion, and insecurity. Trust is not just about being faithful; it's about being reliable, honest, and transparent with your partner. It's about knowing that your spouse has your back, no matter what.

When trust is broken, it can feel like the ground beneath you has shifted. Rebuilding it requires time, patience, and consistent effort. But it's worth it. A marriage rooted in trust allows both partners to feel emotionally, mentally, and physically safe. This safety fosters deeper intimacy and opens the door to vulnerability, which is the lifeblood of a lasting connection.

Every person comes into a relationship with their own set of experiences, fears, and dreams. Understanding your partner means taking the time to learn who they truly are, beyond the surface. It's about listening not just to respond but to comprehend.

Understanding doesn't mean you'll always agree, but it does mean you'll approach disagreements with empathy and respect. It means recognizing that your partner's emotions and perspectives are valid, even if they differ from your own.

Misunderstandings are inevitable in any marriage, but they don't have to be destructive. When both partners prioritize understanding, conflicts become opportunities for growth rather than barriers to connection.

Affection is the glue that binds a couple together. Small gestures like a warm hug, a soft kiss, a kind words, communicate love in ways that words sometimes cannot. Over time, the busyness of life can cause affection to wane, but it's essential to keep it alive.

Affection isn't just physical; it's also emotional. It's showing gratitude for your partner, celebrating their achievements, and supporting them through their struggles. It's the little things like holding hands during a walk, leaving a note on the fridge, or saying "I love you" before bed to remind your spouse they are cherished.

Marriages don't fall apart overnight. Disconnection often begins subtly missed date nights, less physical intimacy, and avoidance of difficult conversations. Early signs of reduced affection and commitment should never be ignored.

If your partner seems distant, stops sharing their thoughts or feelings, or avoids spending time with you, these are signals that something may be amiss. Similarly, if conflicts go unresolved or your partner becomes overly critical or dismissive, it's a sign that your relationship needs attention.

The key is to address these signs early. Open communication is your most powerful tool. Ask your partner how they're feeling, what's been on their mind, and what they need from you. Be willing to listen without defensiveness or judgment. The sooner you address these issues, the easier it will be to resolve them.

Healthy marriages don't just happen; they are built, brick by brick, through intentional effort. Love may be the foundation, but effort is what turns a house into a home. This means prioritizing quality time together, checking in on each other emotionally, and making space for romance and fun.

Intentionality also means being proactive. Don't wait for problems to arise before working on your relationship. Regularly assess how you and your partner are doing. Are you communicating well? Are you meeting each other's emotional and physical needs? Are you aligned with your goals and values?

Marriage is one of the most profound relationships we can experience, and while it requires effort, the rewards are immeasurable. A healthy relationship brings a sense of belonging, emotional support, and joy. It provides a safe space where both partners can grow individually and as a team.

When trust, understanding, and affection are nurtured, a marriage becomes resilient. It can weather life's inevitable storms, from financial stress to health challenges, because the bond between partners is strong.

Reflect on your relationship, ask yourself: Am I doing everything I can to nurture my marriage? If the answer is no, take heart. Every day is a new opportunity to strengthen your connection with your spouse. Small changes can lead to significant improvements over time.

Marriage is not about being perfect; it's about being present. It's about showing up for your partner, even when it's hard. It's about choosing love, forgiveness, and understanding, even when it feels easier to walk away.

If you've identified signs of disconnection in your marriage, don't despair. Acknowledging the problem is the first step toward healing. With openness, effort, and perhaps the guidance of a counselor, lost trust can be rebuilt, affection can be reignited, and understanding can deepen.

Every marriage is unique, but the principles of trust, understanding, and affection are universal. They are the lifelines of a healthy relationship, and when nurtured, they can transform even the most fractured marriages into something beautiful.

Choose to love. Choose to grow. And most importantly, choose each other every single day.